Who Says It's Too Soon

MY FIRST YEAR WITHOUT HIM

THE SECRET DATING DIARIES FROM

MAXINE LYN

WELSTAR PUBLISHING
NEW YORK, NEW YORK

Written by Maxine Lyn Raskin
Published by Welstar Publications, Inc.
Horace Batson, Ph.D., Publisher
628 Lexington Avenue, Brooklyn, NY 11221.
Phone: (646) 409-0340
E-mail: publisher@welstarpublications.com
or drbatson@optonline.net
ISBN: 978-0-938503-90-3

Managing Editor, Laura Koplewicz, Ph.D.
Book Design/Typography, Lori Monroe

DEDICATION

Let me dedicate these diaries to my wonderful daughters Mindy and Heather. They didn't blink an eye reading them. Also, to my son-in-laws, David and Les, who did a bit of blinking with some eye rolling. And finally to my beautiful granddaughters, Renee, Georgia and Rachael, who let me know they thought I was a real cool grandma. Finally, to all my great friends, who always were encouraging and never said, "What? You are too old for this."

As I say in the diary, my husband Arnie is right here with me looking over my shoulder and there is no doubt we are still a team, so this is our dedication.

A NOTE TO THE READER

❖

What you are about to read are my personal dating diaries. I believe they should not be edited, meaning you might find missing periods, run-on-sentences or quotes without apostrophes. I also chose not to tuck them in a drawer, but instead share them, encouraging people to enjoy the single life as I have.

If you choose to date, it can be done all the way into your nineties - whether you are a widow, widower or divorcee. The trick is to stay healthy. And may I say, companionship helps on any level, whether it is the opposite sex or same sex, if that is your preference.

I am still moving forward turning new pages, hopefully into my nineties and beyond. You can too.

~ MAXINE

A FIRST FOREWORD (BY ME)

❖

There is not time to practice for widowhood the first time around, particularly when you are close to 72 years old. The one thing you can do is get a Lifeline type gadget to wear on your wrist and be ready to press it if an emergency occurs. They even have you check it once a month and that's the practice. So, I say get on with a happy life. Happiness and grief can go hand in hand. My forty six year marriage to Arnie was a happy one, with the usual or not so usual bumps in the road, much of it recorded on video. I enjoy watching and will continue to do just that. It makes me feel good, something no one can take away.

Perhaps there are two reasons I started to write about widowhood. First, a friend happened to comment that I seemed like a poster child for positive grieving, making me wonder if something was wrong and maybe I would just fall apart soon, but so far I haven't. Secondly, while having coffee with a long-time widow, she made me realize I was different from her when I asked her how she was now after being a widow for so long. She answered,

"You know how it is", meaning it never got better. My "how it is" already was different from hers, not negative.

And speaking of negative, let me discuss my take on the morbid word, widow. For me it conjures up thoughts of black widow spiders, a widow's walk, and those referring to widows as poor or rich ones. A widow's peak in the center of your hairline is no bargain either. Getting back to widow's walk for those who may not know, it's a balcony surrounding a home overlooking water. In the olden days women would stand there waiting for their husbands to return from a dangerous sailing. Guess what? The men many times would not return. How's that for pleasant? When I mentioned these thoughts to a male friend, he came back with a better expression for a widow," a hot babe who lost her husband too soon". True, most of us don't look like that, but babe sure beats widow. That made me think of pretty dresses and lovely nighties that could certainly help being a hot number.

There is definitely a time to call yourself a widow and that is when you need a favor from a company. Usually you will hear, "I am so sorry for your loss", and perhaps you get something for free or at least a discount.

So, let's begin my exciting journey exploring and navigating through the single experience. My friends and family were great support but at the end of the day when your door closes you are cooking for one and in bed alone or with an animal companion. Some choose to look for another mate, others like myself choose to stay single. But, whatever it is you decide, know that you can go on to a happy and productive life.

A Widow's Thoughts

I cry when I see a bright blue sky

I cry when I've accomplished something
I've never done before

I cry when I unpack my suitcase
in a hotel room alone

I cry because you are not there
to share these joys

But when I realize
you are only a dimension away

I stop crying,
Enjoy the sky, and Finish unpacking

I look forward to the next challenge for me
And continue life, moving forward with a smile.

CHOICE LEADING UP TO A FUNERAL

My next two chapters may not seem positive as the titles include the word funeral, however I feel that it may help others cope better if they encounter a similar situation making life and death decisions for or with a loved one.

After two and a half years of on again off again chemo cocktails, and a few fun trips thrown in with chemo on hold, Arnie ended up in the hospital for many weeks being seen by many doctors other than ours, whom we didn't even know. Even worse they didn't even know what each other knew except for charts, not always kept correctly. All this led to Arnie coming down with Legionnaires Disease and that in the end killed him, not his lymphoma diagnosis. Side effects led to rehab and the day he was to be released to go home, he got a leg blood clot requiring hospitalization again. Depressed and deflated of hope we decided together that if things went too far south, we would choose hospice over suffering. Then a strange Dr came by and began discussing leg surgery. South had arrived.

Home we went to a hospice bed and with my help, administering morphine at assigned times, Arnie passed over peacefully surrounded by friends and family as many times described in news stories. Now what? Decisions still had to be made........for a funeral of course.

THE UPLIFTING FUNERAL

So, can a funeral be uplifting? My answer is a resounding YES. In short order my daughters and I decided to give Arnie a military funeral as he was a proud Marine. The only thing he requested to be on his stone was, " I hope the journey continues". More about that journey in the next chapter.

As it was, Arnie's beautiful plain wooden casket draped in the American flag came into view as taps played. It looked spectacular with trees and mountains in the background. I didn't cry during the ceremony as I was caught up in this beautiful cemetery setting. Maybe when you are on Lorazepam, everything is foggy and unreal, but others expressed that same uplifted feeling. Believe me, there were plenty of tears lined up and waiting for the rest of the year and more. I can't live on drugs forever and function.

Now home for the food festivities which every culture seems to have in common. If it's not meat balls, it may be fried chicken and in our case it was lots of corned beef.

Back to the inscribed stone for Arnie. He was wasn't sure if he believed as I did in afterlife, but as you read on, you may be convinced as my family is, that the journey does continue.

ANOTHER DIMENSION

Here goes.....Arnie's stone says "I hope the journey continues": by now he knows it does and so does my family as well as many others who have had experiences similar to those I am about to describe.

I don't know where else Arnie may be but his spirit is definitely around my family and it became clear that this was not a figment of our imagination or wishful thinking after we attended THE CONCETTA SHOW . Who might you ask is Concetta? She is a well- known medium and author who can demonstrate to an audience how she communicates with spirits in the room. As she explains it, the spirits come to her mind, many at a time with messages for the living who are in the audience. Being able to do this is a gift she discovered in childhood.

My daughters, Mindy and Heather, came along with me hoping Concetta would connect with Arnie somehow. She chooses about thirty people from the audience and when she was up to the thirtieth and we weren't one of them, a strange thing happened.

She stood in front of a woman and said, "Arnie, Arnold, both names used by my husband." Continuing, she named my daughters Mindy and Heather, saying Heather was pregnant. That was the telltale sign. Heather had just found out about her pregnancy a few days before and no one knew except the immediate family.

At that point the women she was directing the message to said that she heard nothing that applied to her. Then Concetta redirected her thoughts to the proper person and spirit. Arnie always persistent in life was again persistent in spirit.

My only explanation was that he wanted Heather to know he was there on some level and busted through all the spirits in her mind to do just that. Unlike Mindy and me, Heather did not believe in the possibility of afterlife. This experience changed her mind. If you are open to communicating with an energy that has passed over, you can have some amazing experiences. Over the years we have had countless ones, but I will just relate the following few examples:

VERY CONVINCING

Psychics will tell you that the spirit can communicate through flicking lights, tipping pictures on the wall, and using metal objects. If asked in question form they can help you find things. The finding situation is important for me because I am constantly losing objects and ninety percent of the time Arnie shows me the way unless I actually lost an object in thrown out garbage. After a while you realize these happenings are not a coincidence. Let me give you another example.

Many of my paintings on the wall become slightly crooked and I fix them thinking this must be a way to show me he is around , but in this one instant there was no doubt. There is a family photo hanging in my office against a space surrounded by thick molding. In order to tip it, you would have to lift it over the molding .As I was on the phone with a friend, my back to the photo, I said something that Arnie would have strongly disagreed with. When I finished the conversation and turned to leave, this photo was over the molding and practically upside down. Even an earthquake couldn't make that happen. Coincidence?

Psychics will also explain that you can have a visit from the other side. It is distinguished from a dream because there is no over lapping of happenings, just a strong sense of the person clearly there with you.

Mindy and I both had a visit right after Arnie died. He came to me in my sleep dressed in nice golf clothes looking handsome and healthy. He jumped on my bed and I said, "I thought you were dead". He smiled at me, I grabbed his leg and then he disappeared. Oddly enough that same night he appeared to Mindy. When we compared outfits, we both described the same one, nothing that he ever had worn in real life. Coincidence? I think not.

And the coincidences keep coming for my daughters and me. It makes for a very interesting existence and some good stories. We have a high awareness Arnie is around us and sometimes when my dog stares at something above her and nothing is there, I wonder if she is seeing or feeling his spirit. Dogs live their lives in Alpha so they may sense this dimension more than we do. This leads me to write about my wonderful, loveable and sometimes naughty dog, Daisy. She came to me in the nick of time or was that part of some kind of plan?

MY DAISY

On my cover

Under my cover

On my sheet

Pushes hard against me

Gives a sigh

Scratches quickly

Stays still and quiet

Morning comes

Feet in the air

Time for a belly rub

Man's best friend

My best friend

My Daisy

NOT A MINIATURE GOLDEN

Ever since I was ten, there was a dog in my life but I never needed or appreciated one more than now. Ok, so Arnie didn't like dogs, but lived with me and whatever dog I had. That was love. I did promise when my last dog died there would be no more. It was not to be.

After Arnie got his lymphoma diagnosis and thought there was not a large window of time left for him, he said I should get another dog for my future. Little did he know he would be living with our new dog Daisy for two and a half years.

She came to us at six weeks of age and is now a wonderful companion. Looking like a miniature golden, (there is no such thing) she is really a mix of Cocker, Papillion, Maltese, Pug and Dachshund. Her daddy jumped the fence.

After chewing up almost everything in my house and eating half of it, I still think she is the most wonderful and loving pet. How about finding her chewing on a dildo thinking it is some kind of vibrating bone.

Nothing is safe from her jaws: her heart worm medicine encapsulated in plastic, rubber as in rubber bands, metal as in pins, razors and paper clips, flowers and what about a total chicken carcass down to the bare plate. So far I have been lucky that she has a strong tummy. Sometimes I think it wasn't an accident that she came to me at the right time giving me loving aggravation and plenty of exercise.

The best is that she jumped into my bed the first night I was alone and has been there every night since.... When I am sobbing with sadness, she jumps on my lap and cries with me, although lately she has been coming and just looking at me as if to say, "We've cried enough." I do love Daisy, but I still would like some company with two legs instead of four, which leads me to those who think this kind of thinking is too soon.

WHO SAYS IT'S TOO SOON

Ok, who's to say I'm not ready, not ready for what? I'm traveling, working, dating, having intimacy, teaching, eating, sleeping and going to the movies.....another words, I do not have to stop living because I am grieving, a natural process that takes me with the flow.

You can get on with life side by side with grief. Five months after Arnie passed, I took a short cruise alone from NY to Bermuda just to see if I could do it. My son-in-law took me to the pier, later telling my daughter who in turn reported to me that he said, "I was like a child going to the first day of Kindergarten, very nervous". So nervous, in fact, that I left my whole purse, money, passport and more on the scanner. Thank heavens for the woman behind me who called my attention to it when I was half way to boarding the ship. Everything went up hill from there.

When my doctor heard I was doing this, there was a very long pause and then the famous words,

"Isn't it too soon?" I sat up looked at him and said this is what I want and need to do. On my way out, he wished me a good journey.

So many people were saying this to me and suggesting grief groups that I finally gave one a chance and ended up helping others, but I didn't need them to deal with my feelings. I was doing just fine......Each to his own.

I traveled to Mohonk Mt house with my children and grandchildren twice, a place Arnie and I loved. It was emotional walking into the room alone and knowing this is it, but I made new memories with my family and continue to love it and will return, perhaps with a male friend. I like male companionship. After all I had 45 wonderful years of it.

My first date from the internet said he thought it was too soon for me to be dating after just four months without Arnie, but he took me to lunch anyway. I guess he thought he should know since he was a psychologist.... wrong.....wrong.... wrong.

My best friends and family were very encouraging about my getting out into the world, including being part of the dating scene. What I did find out is the dating business is not so easy to handle. First, you need a bit of self- confidence, if not a lot.

SOME REINVENTING GOING ON

In any case, you look in the mirror after crying your eyes out and see puffiness here, there, and everywhere, wondering how you are going to be appealing to some guy who doesn't love you, no matter what, like your husband would have.

Well I thought to myself, go out and find a new wardrobe. Guess what? That is costly, but hey I need to reinvent myself so there I was at the biggest department store with a fashion coordinator ready to sell me a wardrobe, but couldn't find anything that fit or if it fit, it didn't look right.

I sat in more than one beautiful dressing room full of crappy expensive clothes for old people. Since then my daughters have found time to help update my closet. Now there is a lot of throwing out to do, but I'm not parting with things that are 40 years old looking better than what was hanging in the dressing room.

It's time for the hair. No grey please. I need a new style that will not be too short so the hair covers side wrinkles and spots, and not too long because I have to manage it and still look presentable. Nail gels keep my crooked fingers looking their best and work for the crooked toes as well.

Exercise is built in when you have to walk your dog. Sometimes I even have to walk around the yard at three in the morning if Daisy decides she needs an extra outing. Then there is dancing in the house and my trusty yoga mat.

It is easy to let the world go by and not keep up with the latest happenings when you are bogged down with paper work, fixing the mistakes you've made with the check book and things of that sort.

To do more reinventing, I am setting time aside to read so I can have a literate discussion with any future date that might come along. Learning new things is also part of reinvention. Finding the correct size light bulb and getting it in, fixing a running toilet, using a wheel barrel to cart in food, or how about draining the kitchen sink with a plunger, yuck.

Then there is letting the spiders eat the flies on a hidden window sill. Every spider I catch goes over there. I discovered that spicy Tabasco sauce chases the cave crickets, but when a huge bee chased me out of the basement, I ran out of the house the bee close behind, a good plan. I guess I have my own reality show, How to Get Along Alone.

So with new clothes, a new hairdo, some intellectual info and survival confidence, I'll be ready for my close up when you are.

ZOOSK SHMOOSK, MIX AND MATCH

Now I am somewhat confident and ready to hit the dating scene where ever it may be. It's a whole new world with a whole new vocabulary that's news to me.

When my mother gave it a try 30 years ago things were a bit different. A personal matchmaker made the effort to find someone for her and there was just one choice, not her type.

Now it's my turn and out of curiosity about internet dating, with hundreds of choices, I went surfing, seeing photos and profiles of various men, wondering what it would be like to actually have a date now.

There is a dating site called Zoosk, another named Plenty of Fish and so many more I couldn't even list them. With names like that you really have to wonder about it all, especially when they brag their site is free and then tell you your responses will go up 230% if you join the upgraded version for an upgraded price... Where do they come up with 230%? Most peculiar of all, which many of them have, is a virtual gift system. You can send pictures of roses, teddy bears, chocolates and so forth, along with your message to a prospective date. It reminds me of kids' stickers, not very grown up.

The time it takes to fill out your profile and then get your pictures posted is unbelievable. It almost leaves no time for dating. I learned how to get my picture on to a site with the help of my savvy daughter, Heather.

You need to find whatever photos you think are complimentary and that isn't so easy, preferably showing what you enjoy doing and definitely be honest with a recent one. I couldn't find any of me in bed. On the other hand, some of the men look downright scary in their tea shirts or holding a cigarette when their profile says they don't smoke.

Yet another scary thing is the whole section on dating tips and how to protect your personal safety. This is a very long section. Finally, I came to the conclusion that I was most comfortable trying out J Date.

The J in J date stands for Jewish. You pay a fee, those sites being the ones with a better reputation, and that is where I began my dating adventure. Not that religion matters, but it is something in common anyway.

I wish there was an I date, "I" standing for Italian. That's because I love Italy and so many Italian men look handsome to me. Meeting someone for a quick coffee there just wouldn't work anyway.

I do question some of the vocabulary men use for finding and attracting someone to message. There must be A jip sheet somewhere because you see the same words over and over such as: Looking for good hearted women, long term, (if they're old already how long term can it be?) A partner in crime didn't do much for me either. And so goes the beginning of my dating journey.

DITZY DATING

After plunking the forty something dollars down to join J Date for a month, and browsing myself silly getting no responses, I decided to cancel the whole thing. That day a message arrived on the site from a psychologist, who shall remain nameless, age 85, but not aged as you many think.

Ok, I held my breath and called the number he E mailed. I suggested meeting for coffee, but he insisted on lunch, so lunch it was. My opening remark was this question: "Is this going to be a session or a regular conversation?" His answer was, "All my conversations are sessions."

During this first date he asked about what I like to read and all the preliminary stuff people ask to find out about one another. I imagine if you do this often enough it becomes tedious. Anyway, after each answer he would comment that what I said fit my personality. Finally at the end of our meal I asked if he had a name for my personality. His answer was,"Ditzy".

Now it is true I have been considered this from time to time, but I did explain that there was a serious side to me as well, which he did recognize but liked the ditzy part the best.

After three dates I discovered his wife of 47 years was a fabulous cook and when he asked me if I would want to cook for him, I declined, saying cooking wasn't my thing. I did make him a fruit salad which we had when he came back to my house for a meditation lesson. That was the last time I heard from him. Maybe he didn't like the fruit salad.

In any case, my next experience on the internet took me to Plenty Of Fish, which is free, so why not give it a try.

PLENTY OF FISH

This title gave me trouble as I am not fond of fish. Not letting that stop me, I went fishing and hooked another psychologist, age 62. I was a bit dubious to meet without a picture, but hey you don't go around picking your friends for looks so I met him at Panera. He paid for lunch and in the end I gave him advice feeling I earned my lunch.

Imagine a guy looking to date when he was already living with a woman whom he said he loved, but wasn't getting his fantasies fulfilled. I, on the other hand, would do for him if I was willing to do the "whatever". I explained that I was not the one for him and suggested he go home and rethink the situation.

My advice was to take his roommate to a sex shop and look at all the paraphernalia, talk about what he wanted and then see if she would go along. He actually thanked me. We never exchanged names. I was glad I parked my car far away from the restaurant, telling him

I was going shopping in a nearby store, which I did, so he couldn't follow me, and that was the end of it, the old Nancy Drew move.

I did get a response from a real cute 28 year old who said he thought I was pretty and age didn't matter. Well, yes it does, so I dropped him off the line. I know there are Cougars, a group of women who seek younger men, but that is not my thing at the moment. Men need to be older than my son-in laws, now in their fifties.

The question is where can I meet suitable single men? I tried going to a singles gathering at the Temple. We gathered alright, in a circle with nametags that reminded me of school days.

It was uncomfortable to say the least and naturally there are many more women than men, with the women looking at the other women to see their competition. No Thank You. Then there was the Widow and Widowers dinner club. After lousy service at a restaurant, with one or two men to twenty women, I stopped that.

The latest plan is just do what I feel like and if I should find someone of interest that would be great. Being out in public at lectures, museums, etc is important for mental stimulation as well. Obviously staying home all the time is not the answer. I'll be square dancing in January and hope I can keep my left and right straight.

Friends and family have been very supportive and extremely helpful whenever I need them and I have found out you just never know when that might be.

NEED A LITTLE HELP FROM FAMILY, FRIENDS AND AN OCCASIONAL STRANGER

It seems everyone has their own lives and when yours falls apart due to losing a mate whom you relied on for almost everything except cooking, cleaning and social schedules, I found my smoke signals going off every two minutes.

At first your friends can't do enough, except there isn't really that much they can help with as many things have to do with private family matters. Both daughters, Mindy and Heather, took over showing me how to do bills and file, plus helped everywhere else that confused me which was pretty much everywhere.

The real twist here was that Arnie gave direct instructions to Mindy to make sure I didn't throw out important things which he felt I'd do. That was my history, so everything had to be filtered through Mindy. Now she has a huge box of filtered garbage that hasn't been gone through yet, and I'm off limits so far,

Running this house and my life is like being a one person corporation, papers going from here to there, perhaps to the shredder, or back into a pile just in case. My to-file-pile is another thing altogether, best described as falling over. This is all after Arnie spent almost a year getting things in order, planning to sit with me and explain, but he was never quite ready to do the explaining and then time ran out.

Arnie managed to leave me a small nest egg, and small is the best description. When faced with a limited amount of money, even I am paying attention to water running, lights on and costs of groceries etc. I never did that before.

For those in the same position there is a government program called PAAD, created to help those with no or low income. You can get prescriptions for no more than $7.00.

I also reversed my mortgage and get a monthly income from the house which helps pay taxes and leaves me a bit for fun. Arnie and I froze our taxes many years ago, a good move which is now handy as taxes increased $5,000. Even though I lay it out, I get the difference back every year. Yay, NJ!

I also applied for help paying gas and electric, a big savings. The thing is you have to fill out forms every year which change, so it is confusing and you just pray yours doesn't get lost in the shuffle. There should be a dance called the government shuffle.

IF IT'S NOT ONE THING IT'S ANOTHER

Besides my kids, grandchildren and son-in-laws, there are numerous others who help for a low fee. Neighbors are there for things like gutters I can't reach, or to carry something heavy that comes along.

Even when you have yearly maintenance done professionally, there is plenty in between that needs fixing especially when Irene visits you. There was definitely trouble in River City with that hurricane, and I was pretty close with the river thing when a good sized pond rose up to the basement stairs. This time my smoke signals were on fire as I cried out for help and my family circled the wagons.

They opened a sewer drain to let the water out, bailed out another part of the basement, swore this would never happen again and I called a plumber to put in a sump pump. For $2000 he did the work and Fema paid for it. There was a lot of paper work attached to that as well.

This all followed in the footsteps of the East Coast Earthquake which some felt strongly, others hardly at all and me, I never felt a thing as I was in my car leaving the Ob-gyn's office. Had I been on the table at the time of the earthquake, I might have thought I was having an orgasm.

And how about the surprise snowstorm in Oct with all the leaves still left on trees causing everything to come down on my lawn and half a tree hit the garage. This called for Lorazepam again. All this was going on five days before a big trip which I had to prepare for with no lights or heat. Well, yes, a flashlight doesn't really count.

My dog Daisy and I slept under four covers, me with a fur coat, hat and gloves while Daisy had her own fur coat. Guess I passed the crisis test because I did leave for the trip even as the insurance adjuster walked around my property taking notes with my daughter Mindy.

I've found various people for the different odd jobs who are more like friends than workman and I'm lucky. Saving a bit here and there means another vacation here or there. And speaking of savings, budgeting for everyday life and unexpected emergencies does have to be a priority.

RATHER PLAY MONOPOLY

So, money plays a big part of life's equation and that's not good for me as I have a math learning disability; this doesn't help very much when you're on your own.

Oh, I know there is help, but in the end I have to keep track of my expenses or else, whereas in the game of monopoly I just have to pass go and collect $200 or turn over a mortgage card and get more money. The game has no balance sheets, spread sheets, check books or bills that look like they came from another planet.

Now, I believe if you look hard enough at your life, you can see some kind of recurring pattern that follows you always. My pattern has to do with money. Others may have recurring love problems, drug problems, work problems or constant trouble with their relationships Mine seems to be the money pattern. Starting as a young child, I always seemed to have enough for my needs but never got near the rich mark.

Even when my parents went through a short rich period, I wasn't aware of it and actually asked my father if he had enough money to send me to college. Laughing he said, "Choose anywhere you wish to go".

I found a finishing school that allowed me to eliminate math and science from my schedule. That continued on to Syracuse where I then majored in radio and TV, so no math again. This money pattern continued into marriage, and now my single state. If I am careful, there may be just enough money till I no longer need it. It might just be my luck that I live to 100 or more and that will call for interesting math on my children's part.

It turns out that as my parents had quite a bit of money for a while, I now appear wealthy because my house, the one I grew up in, is in an impressive neighborhood with lots of mansions around. Better yet, I have mom's mink coat and a lovely diamond ring, along with nice clothes that I bought 20 years ago when Arnie was really doing well for a short time. Fortunately I still fit into them.

Workers who come by to give estimates think I can afford the top of their scale, soon to find out I live in a reversed mortgage house and have the bare minimum to spend or even worse am looking for some freebees.

One of my daughter's friends is in finance and has come to see me numerous times explaining checks and what I can spend using a spread sheet. That sheet scares me more than a horror show, but there is no choice other than to get better at it, no matter what. Another friend is helping me with small investments.

I did what Suze Orman suggested and opened a TD Ameritrade account on line. Looking at it just makes me dizzy, but this friend is so trust worthy he has my code. The family talked me into going on an expensive twelve day European cruise with Joan Hamburg and her listeners from WOR Radio. I'll think about the money spent when I get home, not now.

My plan is to spend more while I am still OK and be frugal a bit later. I'm thinking there is nothing better to get my mind off money than sex and that is where we go from here.....enough about money.

WHAT TO NAME THE SEX CHAPTER...
WHOOPS, I JUST DID

Well really, as you might surmise, this chapter won't be very long. I've not had much time to gather new material. Arnie and I had quite an adventurous, playful, and wonderful sex life for 46 years, but that doesn't count now.

The purpose of including some sex talk is hopefully to help those "hot babes" out there who may feel guilty thinking about sex so early in their loneliness, or simply don't know how to discuss it.

We all know sex is an interesting topic as so much of it is included in books, movies, tv, and magazines etc. In fact, just the other day at a couples' party with best friends, the only single person being me, one of the guys asked if I minded answering a personal question about dating. He asked two questions actually, One about whether I was seeing anyone and secondly if I was going to have a chapter about sex. So there you go.

Anyway, at 71 I would like to think I'm not done with sex and can be somewhat of a "hot babe". The best confidant in this part of my reinvention turned out to be, drum roll please, my GYN.

Four months after I became this "hot babe with a husband who died too soon," I was on the table in that famous position wondering how I was going to approach the sex topic. Before I knew it, my doctor brought it up himself. Now, he is my age, a faithful Catholic, and a highly moral person. Boy, was I surprised when he told me I should not be giving up sex and hoped I would be open to it at the right moment. Pardon the pun.

I did explain it was a long time since I had intercourse with Arnie due to his illness, making it a challenge at my age to find a comfortable fit. He told me not to give up and keep practicing. Well, I'd need to start my own personal house of ill repute to manage that, but then I thought a dildo might do the trick. At first I couldn't pronounce the word as my daughter corrected me from saying "dildoo".

At any rate, I feel that if sex had always been an important part of your married life, it still should be an option for those widows who would like that choice. So, I shall take my doctor's advice and be open to intimacy if it suits me.

Now that this discussion has been addressed, I look forward to continuing my life in the forward position.

EPILOGUE:
NO GOING BACK (ONLY FORWARD)

In the end, the only way back to Arnie are memories, my precious films and tape recordings plus photos all over the house. They temporarily take me to another place, connecting the present to the past and then I refocus on the future. That, I think, is a key to a healthy grieving process, looking to the future with enthusiasm, hope and some plans. I do have a wonderful tape Arnie and I recorded together during a trip to Washington, laughing and joking. Once in a while I play it and laugh all over again.

Now I am looking forward to new adventures, new experiences and meeting new people. It is my own personal reality show. The next big event will be a trip to Europe, sailing the Mediterranean with Joan Hamburg and her listeners from WOR radio.. For now, I guess it's bon Voyage.

PLEASE CONTINUE READING

FOR MY ANSWER TO THOSE WHO TOLD ME

IT'S TOO LATE.

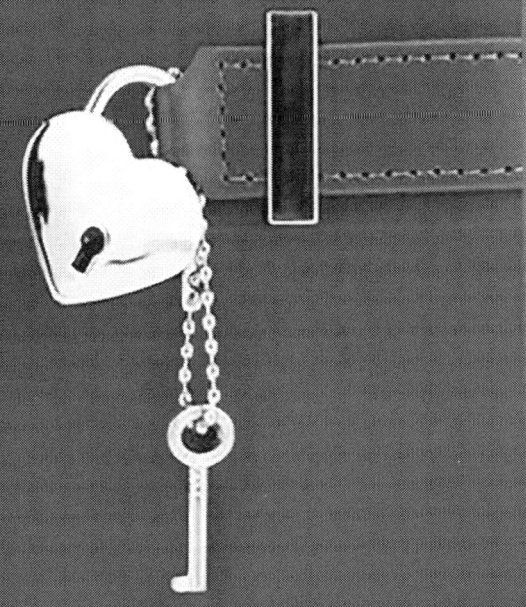

Who Says It's Too Late

ONGOING YEARS

THE SECRET DATING DIARIES FROM

MAXINE LYN

BACK AND FORWARD

80 began in a happy place

With friends, family and my boyfriend, Ace

Now photos spread out on the table

And memories spread out in my head.

Looking backward to knowing then

Looking forward and wondering when.

A SECOND FOREWORD (BY ME)

❖

There is no time to practice for dating except jump right in and smile a lot. Write your profile for the dating sites, perhaps try a bar or two and maybe reach out to friends, letting them know you would like to get fixed up. That's the old fashioned way of saying, "hooked up." I think to myself hook comes from hooker, so think about that one! And let me tell you now, from experience, that bars can be noisy, smoky and most of the time are not worth the eight dollars a drink. Friends are caring, wanting to help, but many can't even manage their own husbands, let alone find you a good match..... so what's left? The internet with endless sites: any sexual preference, any color, any location any financial situation or interests. I did try the millionaire one right off the bat but these guys seem to be looking for statuesque bomb shells and money talks even if the men appear short and stubby. After checking myself out in the mirror I decided to go on to the next possible site. As it is I put my profile on many of them including a cougar one which you will read about later on.

So let's begin looking at my adventures, which by the way, I hope to continue for a long time. One of many role models is Dr. Ruth, now 88, who literally runs from one program interview to the next, a positive example showing you can still be relevant as an OverAge person. And don't forget Sophia Loren, Jane Fonda and the list goes on with me at the end.

So now I consider myself relevant and so do my daughters, granddaughters, son-in-laws and friends. They are impressed that I created a dating reality show based on my dating experiences. I was told people our age aren't marketable. Well, Bachelor is going to do a senior bachelor so now tell me we aren't marketable. I didn't give up. Finally a company in Hollywood asked me to sign a contract allowing them to pitch my show. The contract ran out when nothing happened due to COVID and the fires. Believe it or not right here at home, I got connected to someone who saw my sizzle and wants to coproduce it with me. Here comes my second contract. Not only that, he is pitching it to an interested network.

Now at 81 I will begin telling my stories in the present and work backwards to age 71. The whole idea is for you, the reader, to see it is not too late to add new pages to your life and have some fun doing it, even during COVID.

PEEKABOO (VIRTUALLY)

No explanation is needed for COVID, but because of it many dating sites are inundated with singles wanting to connect from their homes. Now we have temporary virtual dating.

This is virtually not for me but many have jumped in with all sorts of creative ways to meet through the air: making dinners together, zooming, facing, undressing together, playing all sorts of games, texting and even resorting to the phone.

Men and women are lining up potential dates for the future repeating their stories over and over. Some even venture out in masks, staying six feet apart. The surprise comes when the masks come off after restrictions are lifted.

I prefer to tell my stories right here and so I begin with the first one about him.

TAKE A BLACK ACE
FROM THE DECK

So, I met a handsome African American online who lived in Brooklyn and thought I was what he was looking for, someone unconventional. As he was willing to meet me in Jersey I took the plunge and said Ok.

I also admitted to him that I had never dated a black guy. He said I might like it and it turned out I do. We arranged to meet at a nice burger place near my town and I thought I remembered what he looked like. As I was waiting for him to arrive, another African American fellow came in who was not well dressed and frankly a mess with a baseball cap on backwards. My heart sunk. Did I make a mistake?

But that person walked right by me. And at that moment, Ace swooped in with a long stylish coat, tall dark and handsome. I was so relieved I went right up and hugged him and now two and half years later we are still hugging. Ace tells me he really wondered about me being so forward but I did explain. And just to let you know, his real name is Horace, but I said he didn't look like a Horace to me and I asked if he would mind if I called him by the last three letters of his name, ACE, which is much sexier. I guess he didn't mind.

Us

Us we you me

Together
Usweyoume

Sometimes apart
Us We You Me

But always there
A pair

Us we   you me

THE BLACK AND WHITE COOKIE

And speaking of looks, we do make a noticeable couple as many friends have remarked. Ace is quite tall with an athletic build and I am quite small with a petite build. It is not unusual at all for people to remark how much bigger he is than I. Ok, what are they really thinking is our private joke which isn't private any more.

We are different colors, we have different backgrounds and yet we have a lot in common at this point of our lives. We both work on creative projects and encourage one another. But most importantly the chemistry really flies back and forth.

He is ten years younger which makes me a cougar. I read about cougar woman, never thinking I would be one. So you see it's never too late to turn your page and change your ideas. I certainly changed my whole perspective about dating as you will see in the next chapter.

POLYWHATEVER?????

As a married woman for 46 years, being brought up to love, honor and obey just one man and never having strayed during my marriage, can you imagine entering a new world of dating as a widow.

Now I have become a free spirit, loving my independence and not wanting anyone to share my bed or bathroom for more than a few days; that does not count trips.

After many years of this online dating, mostly coffee dates which ended when the coffee was gone, I met Ace, an extremely appealing guy. Right off the bat he let me know that he was not monogamous, believing that you can love or care for more than one person at a time, another words he was polyamorous ; that's a more acceptable name for having your cake and eating it too. Sounded good to me.......

I still loved my husband who is somewhere in the universe so I already was on my way to polyamorousism.

(you won't find that word in the dictionary) Right at the beginning Ace said he wanted to be with me until the wheels fall off. There is a lot of room for that wheel interpretation but I hope they aren't the wheels on his old car.

We see each other every two or three weeks and believe me there is no HO Hum when we do get together. My best male friend, looking out for me, asked what I thought Ace was doing on the weekends we weren't together. My answer was, "I don't care because I am free to do as I please as well."

My whole family and most friends accept the new Maxine. And so the real first date happened that I call the Zipper.

THE ZIPPER

In my opinion the first time you meet someone for a date it is a meeting. If you both decide you want to see each other again, then the first date happens. Ace and I continued passed the meeting to our first date and we're still having dates three years later.

I found out that Ace really enjoys dressing up and going to various places that require a fitting outfit. He expects his date to do the same. Whoops, do I have the clothes for this? Up till now I've been gardening, running local errands, and walking the dog, all in my jeans and sweatshirt.

So, Maxine, now you had better head out and find yourself a sexy dating wardrobe. Speaking of that, Ace has a vision of how he would like to dress me and man-o-man do I love that idea. Why? Because he is willing to buy me some new clothes for playing dress up.

I know some women are rolling their eyes at this point saying this is sexist but I enjoy playing this kind of fantasy game. Besides the fact it saves me some money. Women should be empowered to make themselves happy as they see it, hopefully within reason.

So, what does a zipper have to do with all this? Well for our first date I bought a lovely, tight- sexy dress with a zipper that goes from the top of the dress all the way to the bottom, a new look. The sales gal zipped me up, I loved it and left with my package. Now it is time to dress and wait for Ace except I can't zip the dress.

An SOS went out to my daughter who came right away because I explained it would be first date seduction if he walked in the door and had to do the zipping.

Now fast forward to saying good night. I realized I wasn't going to be able to unzip myself so I waited until he had one foot out the door and I said politely, "By the way, could you just start the zipper for me so I can get out of this dress."

He paused, rolled his eyes and calmly did it, immediately moving down the path and out of sight. When I knew him better I asked what he was thinking while unzipping me and he said ,"I thought Horace, just keep walking".

Walking isn't something Ace can do to get to my house from Bed Stuy in Brooklyn. It can be a two hour trip in traffic especially when they are washing down the

Holland tunnel. His plan is to come very late at night which leads us to the next chapter.

Don't Call The Police!

The path to my home is on a quiet suburban block where not much goes on late at night especially at 3 in the morning. That led me to think it wouldn't be a good idea for my neighbor to glance out her window in the middle of the night only to see a black man emerge from his car and approach my door.

You see Ace and I figured that if he came at that time he would cut out traffic and make the trip quickly without speeding. A black man has to be careful not to speed so he doesn't get stopped. We know how that can play out.

This meant that I needed to chat with my neighbor and forewarn her to the possibility of seeing him and not call the police to save me. This is not the kind of excitement my guest needs.

However she found it all very exciting and passed along the message to her husband so he was aware as well. I knew for sure it wouldn't be long before the whole neighborhood knew about my new social life.

Now that I don't have to worry about the police, I found out Ace does. He is constantly aware, wherever he goes, that he is a "black man in America" as he puts it.

Here's an example: On a hot summer day when he was visiting me wearing a cut off T-shirt and getting ready to go home I noticed him putting on a blazer. I asked him why, as it was so hot and his reply, " I shouldn't drive through the city in a cut off T-shirt which may cause the police to stop me." It would have never crossed my mind. We are constantly learning from one another.

Getting away from serious business, my last story about Ace and me involves a bit of porn. I should have learned my lesson but honestly it happened again.

THE FAMILY PORN STORY
(A FIRST)

When you date on line and many times it is more than one person at a time, text mistakes can occur. My mistake was a doozy that went to my daughter instead of my boyfriend. Most people start their day with a cup of coffee.

I started this particular day with a bang and not the one you may be thinking about. You see my boyfriend and I were doing porn texting early in the morning, having some fun trying to outdo one another as to whom could be more down and dirty.

At five thirty AM, without glasses. I managed to sex text my daughter by accident and once you hit that button there is no return. She couldn't miss it as I had the text punctuated with suggestive, colorful emoji's, not to mention words she never heard from her mother's mouth. I was waiting for the expected phone call which came right away.

My daughter kindly suggested I be more careful after I explained it was a joke. Actually she thought it was funny and suggested I include the incident in my diaries which as you can see I am doing. Even better she had one friend she wanted to tell and of course the rest of the family got filled in as well.

I knew I had an accepting family but this was the best. I also learned it wasn't porn texting, but sexting. Is there a difference?

For many years before I met Ace on line, I collected lots of amusing dating stories, mostly short ones, because the relationships didn't last very long as you will find in the next chapters.

THE LONG AND SHORT OF IT
(MORE STORIES)

The majority of my online dates after the first year without him weren't even dates but chats by phone, E mails or short coffees. I always told dates about research for my show unless I saw a chance for more dates and that almost never happened.

Did I mention that I created a TV dating reality show based on my observations while dating the overage group 65 and up. How many woman meet for a drink or coffee and show up with a pad and pencil. It actually surprised me how many men were open to sharing some of their dating secrets.

ZIPPERS GO BOTH WAYS
(UP AND DOWN)

On a first meeting with a guy, would you tell him his fly is open? Actually using the term fly shows my age group so I will call it his pants' zipper. Either way it was totally down. So now having met with a quick hug which seems to be the going thing to do, before we sat I felt the need to tell him about his senior moment concerning the pants faux pas. He thanked me, zipped up and we had an uneventful coffee.

To spice up the dull conversation I said, "I guess you know where I was looking." And since it seemed neither one of us was going to pursue this meeting further, I suggested WD 40 might keep the zipper going in the right direction. I don't think he found that funny but paid the bill anyway. So there was not magic on this date, but the next one was magical.

ROOSTER STORY
(77 TO 88 OVERNIGHT)

This was an actual date that took place at my home after already having one date that went well. For our second date he suggested coming to my house and cooking an Italian meal for us as he was Italian and called himself a really good cook.

It sounded good to me, hoping he was also good at cleaning up. He arrived holding pots , pans, cooked chicken pieces, jars of Italian sauce and some bread. Put it all together and there wasn't much cooking going on but there was a big saucy mess.

Now get this. Before dessert, which I was providing, and not in the bedroom, I asked him what he was doing heading in that direction. I explained that there was no way I would be off to bed on the second date.

His answer was that I would be missing out because his love making is so wonderful I wouldn't care when he finally told me he was really 88 and not 77 as his profile showed.

I say 77 to 88 overnight is double digit magic and just to let you know, he had a nick name for his cock which was rooster. That certainly was a cockadoodle moment. There appeared, however, a real magical moment in time waiting for me to discover. It was MIPCOM.

WHAT'S A MIPCOM?

Getting married, having a baby and being at MIPCOM were the most exciting things I have ever done in my life and this MIP event happened for me at the age of 77, so go figure. Well, this is the whole point. You can still do exciting and wonderful things later on in life and dating, I discovered, is one of them. I'm getting to MIPCOM.

In the midst of dating, I discovered there's a subculture over 65 that I call over age. These people are dating on all levels including the intimate one, spinning fascinating tales for me to write about.

This gave me the idea for a reality show called Dating Over Age, my project and passion for the past 8 years. It is meant to entertain but at the same time encourage and inspire people, particularly women, to get out there and have fun, while adding a new page to their life. It is permissible. Yes, this is all leading to MIPCOM.

Friends and family will be happy for you, in fact you make their lives easier because you are happier and doing something for yourself instead of totally relying on them.

Finally this brings me to MIPCOM, an acronym for Marche International des Programmes de Communication, much easier to say MIPCOM as you can see. It's a global content event held in Cannes, France where creative people bring their fresh new material to sell.

And there I was along with Kevin, one of my creative partners, hoping someone would love this show idea and pick it up. We navigated through throngs of people, 14 thousand to be exact.

Meetings with networks and production companies were set up ahead at which time I would pull out my treatment page from a bright pink box saying, "out of the box" It had an idea light bulb painted on it, so do you get the idea? At the same time I was wearing a pink badge saying I'm seventy seven and growing up. All this gimmick nonsense was meant to attract attention and be remembered.

Well, something did click as we got some production companies interested enough to request a show sizzle that could be seen on video. Now I had to figure out how to do this mini pilot. OK, I never did something like this before, but, hey, I never wrote a reality show either.

So with the help of many wonderful talented friends and family I found a film maker who turned my house and lawn into a movie set and we filmed the sizzle.

What I really needed was a bunch of straw to turn into gold so I could pay for this or at least some investors. It turned out I was the only investor with a bit of help from my daughter who had faith in me. She was my tech right hand, very much needed as I thought cut and paste on the computer needed glue.

Now the excitement builds. I finally found a co-producer who is pitching my show to major entertainment companies and thinks he can get big bucks for us. I would be happy just getting my investment back, but you can't put a price on the fun I'm having.

Meanwhile, let me begin with a story about a restaurant experience that might sound familiar to you.

You're Not Sitting In A High Chair

This can happen on a first date at any age, but when it happens to an over- age person on a first date, you really have to wonder where they have been most of their life and what are you going to do about a second date.

This is the scenario. He sits across the table from you looking handsome and dapper speaking intelligently and showing a sense of humor; that is one of the most important attributes on a dating profile.

The breakfast of pancakes and bacon is served to you both and don't forget the gooey maple syrup and butter that goes with it. Now he picks up the greasy bacon with his finger, the napkin hiding on his lap and then with no thought to how this looks, he sucks off the mess from all five fingers really enjoying himself and continues this throughout the meal.

At the end with little pancake left, he pushes the end of his meal up on the fork with his finger, totally forgetting there is a knife sitting there ready to be used and does the finger licking good act again.

Well, I think to myself, if he does this, how often does he change his underwear, does he bath and use deodorant often enough, are his sheets on the bed for weeks, are his dishes at home clean along with everything else in his house and so go the thoughts.

Letting all those thoughts go because of a strong chemistry attraction, I chose to have a second date. I am finding out that high chair table manners are a small matter compared to the whole wonderful person. In fact, I find myself picking up the bacon once in a while.

In other words, when you are out there dating, you do need to give the other person a chance. There may very well be something really special under that napkin.

OLDIE BUT GOODIE (AT 92)

There was a chance for me to give a 92 year old a go at it when I thought his profile screamed special. Mr. H, a former Marine, fought in the Second World War and proudly wore a valor medal on his Marine cap. I took notice, as my husband was a Marine as well .There is something special about these guys. So, I met him,

On his profile Mr. H claimed a doctor said he had the body of a 70 year old and I have to admit he looked and acted that way when I met him. To top it off he drove a Jaguar which didn't hurt the cause.

Ok, let's cut to the chase and he did chase me asking that I join him as a companion on an island cruise, already planned and paid for. Are you kidding? It was in five weeks after our first date.

So I turned him down saying I hardly knew him, thinking I could be trapped on a ship with only a life raft. On the other hand my kids thought it was a great opportunity, especially since I was writing about such things and perhaps I would come a away with an interesting story and insight as to what it is like dating someone 20 or more years older.

As a proper female from an upstanding family I suggested we meet each other's families and then gave Mr. H a list of do's and don'ts as to behavior. He accepted the suggestions, and we sailed away in one room with two beds. Our deal was friends without benefits.

I did suggest if we continued our relationship he should find himself a women who gave benefits. He actually did, in fact two of them, in their eighties, although he continued seeing me as we had so much fun together. Mr. H was proud of his sexuality showing you can have a sexual life into your senior years if that is what you choose to do.

Unfortunately after two years and quite a bit of controlling behavior on his part we went our separate ways. His parting words were good bye and have a good life. I did go on to do just that meeting Mr. S, a fellow from India.

"San" Experience

Obviously you need to date in order to collect stories so I kept up a dating schedule. I always would inform my date ahead of time that I was writing a dating diary to eventually be published and asked them if they would help me out by answering questions about their dating experiences .

Now to my San date where, frankly, I felt like a specimen. Let me explain. We met at a restaurant for lunch which was quite generous on his part as we hadn't even met. Sitting across from me before the salad even arrived, his hand found mine, and staring into my eyes he said he was taking me in. That put me on alert right there.

Next he told me he liked my summer dress, that my teeth were nice and white and that my nails were well groomed. All I could think of was, "where's the salad" so I could politely remove my hand from his to grab the fork. He continued on to be romantic but did cooperate answering questions, making sure I knew that if we went on a cruise he would always wear his pajamas at night. I did not ask that question.

He also volunteered his thoughts on friends with benefits which was a must for him but if just friends, the woman pays half. I started to look for my wallet when the check arrived. Actually he paid so I guess his expectations were high for a future date with benefits. There were no benefits because there were no more dates.

As San was younger than me and liking that aspect of it all, I figured why not delve into the unknown Cougar world which is exactly what I did.

COUGARING WITH
"DICK" AND "JOHNSON"

Most of my female friends and even male ones had no idea what a cougar was other than the obvious animal. Neither did I until becoming one, finding out that I enjoy dating younger men who are called cubs. It's not zoo talk, it's sex talk.

There are many sites devoted to this preference and I became part of that zoo culture for research purposes.

Many men actually prefer older women, even women in their eighties. I cannot for the life of me understand why a man would want to be in bed with a wrinkly older woman when they could have a beautiful smooth skinned young one.

The consensus is that an older woman knows what she wants and her maturity is attractive. They also don't have monthly emotional problems. On the other hand, Cougar woman seem to enjoy the youth of a younger man and suggest it makes them feel young.

Sleazy hardly describes most of my experiences on one of these Cougar sites. Along with clothed photos you have the option to request the guy to unlock a button so you can have a peek at him naked at his best. Just like women's boobs, dicks come in all sizes.

To give you an example of how naïve I was, one guy kept referring to the word Johnson which I assumed was his name. Oh No! Later I found out it was another name for his dick. Men's names can be daunting as when you refer to a toilet as a John. Then again, there are probably more names for women's body parts that could fill up a page.

Let's take a look at the choices of men on my cougar site. It seemed as though many of them were not the sharpest knife in the draw. Most were good at texting a few letters together such as NSA, meaning no strings attached and spelled the words a lot as one word.

My profile, unlike many of the women, was not provocative but I still drew some men who found me to be different than the rest. One of them I named BING BANG BOING BOY.

He was 39, thought he was mature, but far from it and agreed to answer my questions about himself as to why he was a cub. It took me a while during our conversation to realize he was busy with himself. He told me later that my voice turned him on. Evidently he was good at multitasking and his ending sound effect was boing. That was enough information for me.

I did date a 40 year old cub who freaked out when he realized I was his mother's age. I have heard that these relationships can work out but during the short experience with him, it was not for either of us.

What I did find out was that I actually preferred younger men, but not 30 years younger. With older men you may have to deal with pills, gadgets to help them sexually and an array of their health issues. I came up with the magic number difference, around ten years. I prefer dirty dancing to the fox trot.

The stories are never ending, but this diary must have an end so I will finish with some thoughts and observations in no particular order.

ENDSAY
(COLLECTED THOUGHTS & OBSERVATIONS)

Over a ten year period I have collected so much material about dating that my desk is covered with it and draws are overflowing with it. Now is the time to write what I feel is pertinent and fill up my recycling bin with the rest. This is the time to concentrate on my show, Dating Over Age, hoping it will not need to be recycled, just replayed for those who need some dating encouragement.

ONE LINERS AND
A LITTLE MORE

"My skin may be wrinkled, but not my soul" (said by Maxine)

When you date allow yourself to mix and match with different cultures. races and religions.....it's fascinating and a great learning experience.

When you take a photo for your dating profile don't take it in the bathroom. Your shower curtain is a dead giveaway-

In a NY Times article about grieving and getting on with it, they wrote, "You can honor your past, but don't have to live in it. People have an endless capacity to love".

Whatever your preference is in relationships, vanilla or different flavors, go for it.

Songs are a great way to communicate. They may say what you are too shy to express.

You are never too old to role play in the bedroom, but you might prefer doing it in the dark.

Someone wrote," You can fall in love with the most

unexpected person in the most unexpected place."

Fun and sex are both three letter words that can mean the same thing. Watch it when a profile says let's have some fun.

I would describe serial-hook- up dating as a string of honeymoons.

I say you can't get arrested for being Over Age. That's a benefit.

If someone on line that you want to date is suspicious but you are still curious and want to meet him, suggest he meet you at the police station.

A Few More Tidbits

A very common expression used by men on dating sites is, "Looking for a partner in crime". Excuse me, I don't want to end up in jail.

Beware when you read the description saying they have a few extra pounds. A few could be an extra hundred.

Would you believe that some widows check out the obits to find a widower who they can visit with a pot roast in hand as an introduction.

I saw a sign I liked in a restaurant saying, "The best stories are not told over a salad". It hung over a bar.

Should an older senior really write down that he is looking for a life partner? Maybe it is handy to have someone monitoring your pill box.

If she wears sup hose under her bathing suit, you can bet they're not married.

A senior female friend of mine said that dating is a great motivator to take a bath, get dressed up, and not wear Carters underwear.

When they can't put a subject and predicate in the same sentence, that's not a good sign.

The ABC's of texting: NSA, no strings attached, sounds like a government program. Seniors know NBC and CBS but they should also know about STD's. You can Google the list of text letter combinations if you want to understand many of the younger daters who use this language. It helps you communicate with your grandkids as well.

One of the more astute guys told me, "An older woman can have the joy of a younger man if she can handle it". There is truth to that with the help of estrogen, coconut oil and a tube of lube.

WHERE DO I GO FROM HERE?

Where do I go from here? To Dating Overage of course. My diaries have been the inspiration for this show and now the marketing and programming people have caught up to me.

They are realizing that our age group of 65 and over can be fascinating and a money making proposition. The proof is that ABC is going to do a Senior Bachelor. Am I going to give a rose? Maybe not, but something tells me I will need to buy another diary.

And Dear Diary, may I leave you with this thought: Going on a date is like reading a book, a live talking book. You learn so much......Just make it a good book.

ACKNOWLEDGMENTS

Many thanks to my publisher, Dr. Horace Batson, for his wonderful patience, encouragement and humor as he helped to make this book idea a reality. I also wish to thank Dr. Laura Koplewicz for her thoughtful manuscript guidance, and to Lori Monroe for her creative magic designing my cover. Finally thanks to my wonderful daughter, Heather, who greatly helped me with double checking my words and making sense of everything on the computer.

ABOUT THE AUTHOR

Maxine is living life happily with her family nearby, enjoying her social life as she grows up and looks forward to keeping those pages turned. Her dog Daisy watches over the house as Maxine pursues a new career based on the show she created, Dating Over Age. The object of this show is to encourage others to turn a page in their lives and find happiness as well.

Made in the USA
Middletown, DE
24 October 2021